The Art of Relaxation: Enhancing Work Efficiency with Yoga Techniques

Author
Aria Shelley

Table of Content

Chapter 1:
Introduction

Sustaining maximum productivity and efficiency is crucial for success in today's demanding and fast-paced work situations. In the middle of the chaos, people frequently struggle with stress, weariness, and mental fatigue, which can seriously impair their capacity to function at their best. The incorporation of yoga techniques into the workplace offers a comprehensive solution that not only solves these issues but also fosters a state of balance, concentration, and wellbeing.

Yoga is a traditional Indian form of exercise that provides a holistic approach to improving mental and physical wellness. Its wide range of practices, which include meditation, mindful movement (asana), and breath work (pranayama), have been shown in studies to lower stress, boost vitality, and enhance attention. People can access a multitude of advantages that directly contribute to increased productivity and effectiveness at work by adopting these habits into their daily routine.

The context for investigating the relationship between yoga poses and productivity at work is established by this introduction. We will explore the specific yoga practices and philosophies that can be easily incorporated into the contemporary workplace throughout this talk. Each approach offers a useful way to improve attention, control stress, and create an environment that is conducive to maximum productivity. These range from basic breathing exercises to restorative stretches and mindfulness activities. Incorporating yoga's wisdom into the workplace has the potential to improve employee performance while also fostering an environment that promotes success and well-being.

Chapter 2:

Evening Elegance:
Prelude to Peaceful Sleep

Evening Style:
The Lead-Up to Restful Sleep

It's getting more and harder to find peace and quiet before bed in the hectic world of modern living. However, the night presents a special chance to establish an elegant ritual—a preface that leads us into a restful sleep. "Evening Elegance" is more than just a slogan; it's a way of thinking that invites us to rethink how we end the day and prepares us for a refreshing sleep.

The Value of Evening Customs

Our nights frequently act as a link between the calm of the night and the bustle of the day. Creating an elegant nighttime ritual is not just a luxury, but also essential to our general health. Acknowledging the importance

Components of a Classy Evening

1. **Mindful Transition:**
 Leaving the hustle and bustle of the day behind and entering the calm of the evening is the first step toward evening elegance. To prepare the mind for a mental shift toward relaxation, this may entail a few minutes of mindfulness during which one considers the day's successes and difficulties.

2. Digital Detox: It's important to cut off from digital gadgets as the evening wears on. The gentle illumination of screens tampers with the body's innate circadian cycle, upsetting the synthesis of the hormone that promotes sleep, melatonin. A sophisticated evening substitutes more calming, analog activities for screen time.

3. Calm Ambience: Establish a setting that promotes serenity. Use soft, warm-toned lighting, light a few candles, or turn down the lights. The body gets ready for sleep when the sight changes to a softer ambience, which tells the brain it's time to wind down.

4. Calm Activities: Take part in calm activities instead than stimulating ones. Ideal activities can include taking a slow stroll, doing moderate yoga, or reading a book. These pastimes not only promote relaxation but also operate as a link between the hectic pace of the day and the peacefulness of the night.

5. Nutrition and Hydration: Eating dinner mindfully might help create a calmer evening. Choose herbal drinks and small, easily digested foods. It is best to avoid large meals right before bed to avoid pain .

6. Reflective Practices: Including activities that encourage introspection, such journaling or thankfulness exercises, in the nightly routine can help people feel wrapped up. Thinking back on the good things that happened during the day helps one maintain an optimistic outlook, which lowers stress and improves emotional health.

Exposing the Technique of Evening Magnificence

Developing a Ritualistic Method:
Nighttime grace is nourished by regularity. The foundation of a calm before-bed routine can be the establishment of a regular and customized ritual. A sequence of relaxing exercises that inform the body and mind when it is time to change from day to night may be a part of this ritual.
Start by determining the pursuits that personally speak to you. This could be taking a few minutes to meditate, taking a warm bath with soothing essential oils, or just sipping on a cup of

Accepting Slow Living: Adopting the concepts of slow living becomes crucial in the pursuit of evening elegance. A methodical and thoughtful attitude to daily tasks is promoted by slow living, which places an emphasis on quality rather than quantity. When applied to the evening, this concept invites us to appreciate every second of the time, be it a peaceful discussion, a leisurely walk, or the simple task of making a warm beverage.

The Power of Aesthetic Surroundings: Our surroundings' aesthetic qualities have a significant impact on how we feel mentally. The setting must be carefully chosen for evening elegance in order to generate sentiments of peace and tranquility. Purchasing plush furniture, soothing color schemes, or sentimental artwork that embodies the idea of tranquility are all worthwhile investments.

Mindful Movement: Including simple movement exercises in the nightly regimen helps to harmonize the body and mind in preparation for sleep. Particularly yoga stands out as an effective method for relaxation. A series of calming, gentle positions can help relieve stress that has built up during the day, leading to both physical and mental relaxation.

Building Connection: Developing elegance for the evening may be a group activity as well as an individual one. Spend time with those you love and cherish by doing things that make you feel close and at ease. A shared dinner, a peaceful stroll, or a private time spent together, the shared goal of evening sophistication can improve the general standard of sleep in a shared area.

Scientific Understanding of Evening Beauty

Evening grace fits in perfectly with our scientific understanding of circadian cycles and sleep hygiene. Our bodies naturally release melatonin as the day wears on, indicating when sleep is about to begin. External variables, such exposure to strong lights and computer screens, can obstruct this process, though. Evening elegance is in line with our circadian rhythm, allowing for a more seamless transition into sound sleep with its emphasis on low lighting and digital detox.
Moreover, the parasympathetic nervous system is stimulated by the relaxing practices linked to evening elegance, such mindfulness and gentle movement. This activation promotes a relaxed state that is beneficial to sleep by counteracting the stress response.

Recognizing the Effect on the Quality of Sleep

Embracing nighttime elegance is not only a romantic idea; it's a useful investment in your general health and quality of sleep. Good sleep has been linked in numerous studies to enhanced emotional stability, physical well-being, and cognitive performance. By deliberately developing a sophisticated nighttime routine, people are not only establishing a calm transition to slumber but also building the groundwork for a more active and full existence.

Useful Advice for Adopting Evening Elegance

1. Establish a Customized Ritual:
Decide which things make you happy and establish a customary nighttime routine. This could involve a mix of relaxing activities like reading, stretching, or meditation.

2. Establish Consistency:
Evening elegance works best when there is consistency. Create a schedule and make an effort to follow it so that your body and mind can learn when it's time for bed.

3. Establish a Calm Environment:
Take note of how beautiful your surroundings are. Use cozy furniture, soothing color palettes, and soft lighting to create a tranquil atmosphere.

4. Digital Detox:
Set aside a certain amount of time each evening to avoid using electronics. With this digital detox, blue light interference is removed from your brain, allowing it to relax.

5. Mindful Movement: Make mindful movement exercises a part of your nightly regimen. This might be a quick yoga practice, a contemplative stroll, or even just some tension-relieving stretches.

6. Develop Relationships: If at all feasible, involve loved ones in your quest for evening elegance. Collaborating in peaceful pursuits with one another cultivates a feeling of unity and peacefulness.

Resolving to Accept the Calm of Evening Elegance

The search of evening elegance appears as a counterweight in a culture that frequently exalts work and nonstop activity—a deliberate welcome calm and make room for sound sleep. The evening's elegance is found in simplicity, decision to attentiveness, and a purposeful slowing down rather than in excess.
Let's not undervalue the opportunity for change that exists in the evenings while we manage the responsibilities of everyday life. By adding grace to our evenings, we develop a close relationship with our own health.

Chapter 3:

Breathe full Bliss:
Yoga's Gateway to Tranquility

Within the chaotic embroidered artwork of advanced life, where stretch is frequently an unwelcome companion, the old hone of yoga rises as a relieving analgesic, advertising a portal to tranquility through breath full delight. Established in centuries-old shrewdness, yoga isn't fair a physical work out but an all-encompassing approach to well-being, welcoming people to investigate the profound connection between breath, body, and intellect. Within the tender stream of asana and the musical grasp of cognizant breathing, specialists discover a way that leads to a peaceful and serene state of being.

At the heart of yoga's transformative control lies the breath □"an unpretentious however powerful constrain that joins the physical and the supernatural. Breath full euphoria, as experienced through yoga, may be a state where each inhale and breathe out gets to be a conscious act, a careful travel into the show minute. The breath, frequently neglected within the hustle of way of, life gets to be a direct, delicately driving specialist to a domain of inward calm and adjust.

Yoga's accentuation on cognizant breathing isn't a unimportant detail; it could be a foundation of the hone. The musical inward breath and exhalation act as a bridge between the outside world and the inside scene. In each breath, there's an opportunity to discharge pressure, let go of diversions, and adjust the intellect to the unpretentious rhythms of the body. As the breath extends, so does the association to a quiet internal space.

The **physical stances**, or asana, in yoga are planned not as it were to improve adaptability and strength but too to encourage a developing mindfulness of the breath. Each movement is synchronized with inward breaths and exhalations, making a liquid move that energizes a thoughtful center. As the body streams through the arrangements, the breath gets to be a grapple, establishing specialists within the show and cultivating a sense of mindfulness.

One of the foremost crucial viewpoints of yoga is pranayama "the cognizant control of the breath. Through various pranayama methods, people learn to tackle the life drive within the breath, developing a sense of adjust and essentialness. Strategies such as Ujjayi, the triumphant breath, and Nadi Shoshana, interchange nostril breathing, direct specialists into a space of profound calm, advancing mental clarity and enthusiastic balance.

Breath full euphoria isn't kept to the yoga tangle; it expands into life style . The mindfulness developed through yoga saturates the way people approach challenges, lock in with others, and explore the complexities of the present day world. The capacity to tap into a peaceful state of being, secured by the breath, gets to be an important apparatus in overseeing stretch and cultivating enthusiastic versatility.

The hone of yoga isn't a one-size-fits-all endeavor; it could be an individual travel that adjusts to the interesting needs of each person. For a few, the energetic vitality of a Vanesa stream may be the door to breath full euphoria, whereas for others, the stillness of a Yin yoga hone may offer a more profound association. The magnificence of yoga lies in its flexibility, obliging professionals of all ages, capacities, and strolls of life. Past the physical and breath-centered viewpoints, yoga envelops a wealthy embroidered artwork of reasoning and morals that advance contribute to its transformative control. The Yama's and Naima's, moral guidelines outlined in classical yoga logic, serve as a compass for cognizant living. Specialists are empowered to develop ethics such as non-violence, honesty, and satisfaction, making an agreeable establishment for a life of tranquility.

Within the advanced setting, where the requests of work, connections, and innovation frequently drag people in numerous headings, the need for a haven of tranquility gets to be progressively crucial. Yoga, with its accentuation on breath full euphoria, gets to be not fair a physical hone but a holistic way of life choice. It is an asylum where people can withdraw to discover comfort, revive their spirits, and rediscover a sense of inward peace.

The science behind yoga's effect on the nervous system provides advance bits of knowledge into its capacity to actuate tranquility. The parasympathetic anxious framework, regularly alluded to as the "rest and process" framework, is actuated amid the practice of yoga. As the breath develops and the body unwinds into stances, a cascade of physiological reactions happens, neutralizing the stress-induced actuation of the thoughtful nervous system. The result may be a sense of calm, adjust, and restoration.

In a world where the interest of outside victory frequently takes priority, the hone of yoga welcomes people to rethink their understanding of accomplishment. Past the honors and achievements, yoga emphasizes the significance of inward well-being. Breath full rapture gets to be an indicator of victory, with professionals measuring their accomplishments in minutes of peace, mindfulness, and self-discovery.

The community aspect of yoga encourage improves its transformative potential. Whether practiced in a studio, a community center, or for all intents and purposes, the collective vitality created amid a yoga session makes a steady and elevating environment. Shared breath, synchronized development, and a collective deliberate to discover tranquility weave an embroidered artwork of solidarity among professionals. The sense of association expands past the physical space, cultivating a worldwide community bound by a shared commitment to well-being.

As yoga proceeds to gain popularity, investigate into its physiological and mental benefits has thrived. Thinks about reliably highlight the positive affect of yoga on stretch decrease, mental wellbeing, and generally quality of life. The antiquated shrewdness of yoga finds approval in cutting edge science, advertising a bridge between convention and evidence-based well-being practices.

The travel into breath full delight through yoga could be an energetic and advancing handle. It is not a goal but a ceaseless investigation of the self. Each hone, each breath, gets to be a venturing stone on the way to tranquility. The mindfulness developed on the tangle steadily leaks into the texture of life style, changing challenges into openings for development and developing an attitude of appreciation and acknowledgment.

Conclusion

 yoga stands as an ageless gateway to tranquility through breath full rapture. It is a all-encompassing

hone that rises above the physical, advertising a
significant association between the body, breath,

Chapter 4:
Corporate Zen:
Yoga Retreats for the Working Mind
Introduction:

In the speedy corporate world, where stress and burnout are common, an arising pattern is picking up speed to bring equilibrium and prosperity into the existences of working experts - Corporate Yoga Retreats. With an end goal to cultivate a better workplace and address the psychological and actual difficulties of the cutting edge labor force, organizations are progressively going to yoga withdraws as a way to advance representative prosperity, care, and efficiency.

The Corporate Wellbeing Basic:

The corporate scene has developed emphatically lately, with an expanded spotlight on representative prosperity. Managers perceive the immediate connection between the psychological and actual wellbeing of their labor force and generally efficiency. Accordingly, corporate health programs have become fundamental parts of authoritative systems to draw in and hold top ability. Yoga withdraws, with their all-encompassing way to deal with prosperity, have arisen as a remarkable and successful method for tending to the multi-layered difficulties looked by the cutting edge working brain.

Yoga as an Answer:

Yoga, an old work on starting from India, includes an all-encompassing way to deal with physical, mental, and profound prosperity. Its advantages, which incorporate pressure decrease, expanded adaptability, upgraded center, and worked on close to home equilibrium; make it an optimal answer for the requests of the corporate world. By coordinating yoga into the work environment through withdraws, organizations intend to establish a climate that sustains both the individual and the aggregate emotional wellness of their representatives.

The Ascent of Corporate Yoga Retreats:
Corporate yoga withdraws are not generally restricted to specialty or elective work environments. Large companies, spreading over businesses from innovation to fund, are perceiving the benefit of putting resources into the psychological and actual wellbeing of their workers. These retreats commonly include a mix of yoga meetings, care rehearses, group building activities, and open doors for individual reflection. The objective is to give representatives a restoring experience that furnishes them with the devices to oversee pressure and further develop their general prosperity.

Advantages of Corporate Yoga Retreats:

Stress Decrease:
One of the essential advantages of yoga withdraws is pressure decrease. The act of yoga, joined with the tranquil climate of a retreat, permits representatives to loosen up and deliver collected pressure. This, thusly, adds to worked on mental lucidity and concentration after getting back to the work environment.

Worked on Actual Wellbeing:
Inactive work area occupations can negatively affect actual wellbeing. Corporate yoga withdraws support development and actual work, advancing better stance, adaptability, and in general wellness. These advantages

not just add to the prosperity of the individual yet in addition decrease the probability of business related wounds and medical problems.

Upgraded Group Building:
Yoga withdraws give a novel setting to group building and cultivating a feeling of fellowship among representatives. Bunch exercises and shared encounters during the retreat make bonds that can decidedly affect cooperation and coordinated effort in the work environment.

Expanded Efficiency:
A revived psyche is a more useful brain. By offering workers the chance to re-energize through yoga withdraws, organizations are putting resources into expanded efficiency. Representatives getting back from a retreat are much of the time more engaged, imaginative, and empowered, prompting further developed execution in their expert jobs.

Care and Close to home Equilibrium:
Yoga underlines care and the association between the brain and body. Through contemplation and breathing activities, representatives figure out how to deal with their feelings and develop a feeling of internal equilibrium. This advantages their work as well as adds to an agreeable work environment climate.

Executing Corporate Yoga Retreats:
The effective execution of corporate yoga withdraws requires smart preparation and thought. Here are key stages for organizations hoping to integrate these retreats into their wellbeing drives:

Evaluating Representative Interest:
Prior to sorting out a yoga retreat, it's vital for measure worker interest. Studies, center gatherings, or casual conversations can give significant bits of knowledge into the inclinations and necessities of the labor force.

Picking the Right Scene:
Choosing a suitable scene is significant for the outcome of a yoga retreat. In a perfect world, the area ought to offer a tranquil and normal setting helpful for unwinding and contemplation.

Teaming up with Experienced Educators:
Drawing in experienced and guaranteed yoga educators is fundamental to guarantee the quality and viability of the retreat. Teachers ought to be gifted in adjusting practices to different ability levels and taking special care of assorted needs.

Making a Fair Program:
A balanced program ought to incorporate a blend of yoga meetings, care rehearses, group building exercises, and potential open doors for individual reflection. Assortment guarantees that members get a complete health experience.

Giving Adaptability and Inclusivity:
Perceiving that people have various inclinations and capacities, it's essential to offer an assortment of yoga styles and exercises. This inclusivity permits members to fit their experience to suit their solace levels.

Offering Proceeded with Help:
The advantages of a yoga retreat can reach out past the actual occasion. Organizations ought to consider

offering progressing help, for example, on location yoga classes, care studios, or assets to urge representatives to integrate these practices into their day to day routines.

Contextual analyses:
Organizations Embracing Corporate Yoga Retreats

Google:
The tech monster is famous for its imaginative way to deal with worker prosperity. Google integrates yoga withdraws into its health drives, offering representatives the chance to go to off-site withdraws zeroed in on care, stress decrease, and group building.

Salesforce:
Salesforce, a forerunner in distributed computing, has coordinated yoga withdraws into its corporate wellbeing program. These retreats stress the organization's obligation to worker joy and all-encompassing prosperity.

Patagonia:
Known for its obligation to natural manageability and worker government assistance, open air clothing organization Patagonia consistently coordinates yoga withdraws for its staff. These retreats frequently happen in beautiful areas, lining up with the organization's ethos of association with nature.

Conclusion:
Corporate yoga withdraws address a groundbreaking way to deal with tending to the difficulties looked by the cutting edge labor force. As the corporate world progressively perceives the significance of

representative prosperity, these retreats are turning into a staple in hierarchical health programs. By putting resources into the physical, mental, and close to home soundness of their representatives, organizations are encouraging a more sure workplace as well as receiving the rewards of a more engaged, useful, and connected with labor force. As the corporate Harmony development keeps on developing, it remains as a demonstration of the developing needs of the cutting edge work environment, where the quest for progress is blended with the quest for prosperity.
Is this discussion supportive up to this point?

Chapter 5:
Digital Detox Dusk:
Unplugging for Better Sleep

Introduction:

In a period overwhelmed by computerized gadgets and consistent availability, the significance of value rest has become more articulated than any other time in recent memory. The inescapable utilization of cell phones, tablets, and PCs has penetrated our sleep time schedules, adversely influencing rest examples and generally speaking prosperity. The idea of a "Computerized Detox Nightfall" is building up some decent momentum as people perceive the need to turn off from their gadgets at night to cultivate better rest. This article investigates the connection between innovation use before sleep time and rest quality, the advantages of a computerized detox sunset, and down to earth techniques to execute this fundamental practice for a more tranquil night's rest.

The Computerized Situation:

As innovation keeps on propelling, the commonness of advanced separates our regular routines has become practically pervasive. Cell phones, tablets, PCs, and TVs are essential to work, correspondence, and amusement. In any case, the blue light discharged by these gadgets can impede the body's regular circadian cadence, smothering melatonin creation, the chemical answerable for managing rest. The subsequent disturbance in rest wake cycles can prompt hardships nodding off and a lessening in the general nature of rest.

The Effect on Rest Quality:
The blue light radiated by electronic gadgets is especially tricky at night as it impersonates normal sunlight, indicating to the mind that it is daytime. This impedance with the body's inward clock can prompt deferred melatonin discharge, making it moving for people to slow down and nod off at a sensible hour. The habit-forming nature of web-based entertainment, messages, and online substance can likewise add to a defer in sleep time as people end up engaged in the computerized world as opposed to planning for rest. Moreover, the consistent openness to invigorating substance and warnings can instigate pressure and tension, further compromising the capacity to accomplish a tranquil night's rest. The aggregate effect of insufficient rest on physical and psychological well-being is factual, with connections to expanded hazard of persistent circumstances, disabled mental capability, and compromised safe capability.

Grasping the Circadian Mood:
The circadian beat, frequently alluded to as the body's interior clock, and manages different physiological cycles, including the rest wake cycle. Openness to normal light during the day synchronizes this beat, advancing sharpness and attentiveness. On the other hand, at night, the shortfall of light signals the body to deliver melatonin, advancing unwinding and setting up the body for rest.
The presentation of fake light sources, especially the blue light discharged by electronic gadgets, upsets this fragile equilibrium. By perceiving the effect of computerized gadgets on the circadian mood, people

can find proactive ways to make an advanced detox nightfall schedule that supports better rest.

Advantages of Computerized Detox Sunset:

Further developed Rest Quality:
The essential advantage of taking on a computerized detox sunset is an improvement in rest quality. By limiting openness to blue light and advanced boosts at night, people can upgrade their capacity to nod off quicker and appreciate further, more helpful rest.

Upgraded Circadian Cadence:
Making computerized detox sunset routine aides in lining up with the body's regular circadian cadence. This arrangement upholds the legitimate arrival of melatonin, indicating to the body that now is the right time to slow down and plan for rest.

Diminished Pressure and Tension:
Disengaging from computerized gadgets at night can diminish openness to upsetting or invigorating substance, assisting with mitigating pressure and nervousness. This, thusly, adds to a more loosened up perspective helpful for rest.

Expanded Efficiency and Concentration:
Satisfactory and quality rest is fundamental for mental capability and efficiency. By focusing on rest through computerized detox nightfall, people can encounter uplifted center, further developed memory, and in general better mental execution.

Improved Prosperity:

Reliably rehearsing computerized detox nightfall advances in general prosperity by encouraging better rest propensities. Further developed rest has broad consequences for actual wellbeing, mental versatility, and close to home equilibrium.

Methodologies for Carrying out Computerized Detox Sunset:

Laying out a Steady Sleep time Schedule:
Making a sleep time routine signs to the body that now is the ideal time to slow down. Incorporate exercises like perusing a book, rehearsing unwinding strategies, or participating in delicate extending works out.

Setting Gadget Free Zones:
Assign explicit region of the home, like the room, as gadget free zones. This establishes a favorable rest climate and forestalls the impulse to involve electronic gadgets in the hour paving the way to sleep time.

Actuating Night Mode:
Numerous gadgets currently come furnished with a "Night Mode" or "Blue Light Channel" include. Enacting this mode at night diminishes how much blue light discharged, limiting its effect on melatonin creation.

Laying out Screen Curfews:
Set a particular time each night to shut down electronic gadgets. This lays out a reasonable limit between screen time and sleep time, permitting the body to progress into a condition of unwinding normally.

Settling on Low-Tech Other options:

Supplant advanced exercises with low-tech choices at night. Think about perusing an actual book, rehearsing care reflection, or taking part in quieting exercises that don't include screens.

Imparting Limits:

Impart the significance of computerized detox nightfall to relatives or flat mates. Laying out a common obligation to turning off at night can establish a steady climate for better rest propensities.

Conclusion:

In the mission for worked on prosperity and generally wellbeing, it is vital to focus on quality rest. The reception of a computerized detox sunset fills in as a proactive and reasonable way to deal with relieves the adverse consequence of innovation on rest designs. By perceiving the significance of lining up with the body's normal circadian mood and executing procedures to decrease evening screen time, people can encounter the significant advantages of better rest. Embracing a computerized detox sunset isn't simply a direction for living; it is a cognizant interest in one's wellbeing, essentialness, and generally personal satisfaction.

Chapter 6:

Moonlit Mindfulness:
Embracing Nighttime Stillness
Presentation:

Within the hustle and haste of present day life, finding minutes of stillness and tranquility can be a challenge. However, as the day moves into night, a one of a kind opportunity emerges for mindfulness and reflection. "Moonlit Mindfulness" typifies the thought of grasping nighttime stillness to cultivate a more profound association with oneself and the world. This article dives into the noteworthiness of nighttime mindfulness, the advantageous relationship between the moon and mindfulness, and down to earth ways people can develop a sense of calm and nearness amid the night.

The Nighttime Canvas:

As the sun sets and obscurity covers the world, the canvas of the night sky unfurls, uncovering the moon and stars. For centuries, the night has held a certain persona and appeal, motivating artists, rationalists, and searchers to explore its profundities. Within the domain of mindfulness, the nighttime presents a one of a kind opportunity for introspection and a association with the display minute that's unmistakable from the sunshine hours.

The Moon's Impact on Mindfulness:

The moon, with its tender shine and ever-changing stages, has long been a image of reflection, cycles, and change. In numerous societies, the moon is related with the female, instinct, and the intuitive intellect. Joining the moon into mindfulness hones can extend the sense of association to the characteristic world and upgrade the by and large encounter of stillness.

Lunar Contemplation:
Locks in in lunar reflection amid the nighttime permits people to adjust their mindfulness with the stages of the moon. Whether it's the quiet full moon or the calm class of a bow moon, centering on lunar vitality can bring a sense of quietness and adjust to the hone of mindfulness.

Night Sky Thought:
Looking at the night sky gives an endless and awe-inspiring scenery for thought. The stars, planets, and the moon itself can serve as stays for mindfulness, inviting individuals to let go of day by day concerns and submerge themselves within the breadth of the universe.

Moonlit Strolls:
Taking a careful walk beneath the moonlight offers a one of a kind tangible involvement. The cool night discusses the delicate shine of the moon, and the cadenced cadence of strides makes a concordant environment for reflection and mindfulness.

The Control of Nighttime Stillness:

Calming the Intellect:
Nighttime intrinsically energizes a abating down of exercises. Grasping this natural cadence permits the intellect to quieten, shedding the buildup of the day's busyness. Within the stillness of the night, people can develop a sense of mental calmness and clarity.

Developing Nearness:
The nonappearance of sunshine diversions permits for an increased sense of nearness. Mindfulness amid the nighttime includes completely locks in with one's environment, sensations, and contemplations without the regular daytime boosts. This increased mindfulness can lead to a more profound understanding of the self and the show minute.

Interfacing with Nature:
The night carries a one of a kind vitality, with nighttime sounds, cool breezes, and the delicate gleam of moonlight contributing to a quiet environment. By tuning into these normal components, people can cultivate a significant association with nature, advancing a sense of interconnecting and mindfulness.

Viable Tips for Moonlit Mindfulness:

Make a Nighttime Custom:
Setting up a straightforward nighttime custom can flag to the intellect that it's time to move into a state of mindfulness. This may incorporate darkening lights, planning warm refreshment, or locks in in some minutes of tender extending or yoga.

Careful Breathing beneath the Moon:
Discover a comfortable spot outside, ideally beneath the moonlight. Hone careful breathing, centering on the inward breath and exhalation. Permit the musical design of your breath to harmonize with the quietude of the night.

Journaling by Moonlight:

Set aside a couple of minutes each night for intelligent journaling. Compose down contemplations, sentiments, or appreciation expressions beneath the moonlit sky. The act of putting write to paper can develop the association to internal contemplations and feelings.

Stargazing Contemplation:
Lie down or sit comfortably, look at the stars, and permit your intellect to meander among the groups of stars. This stargazing contemplation empowers a sense of wonderment and ponders, cultivating a careful appreciation for the endlessness of the universe.

Innovation Detox Some time recently Bed:
Grasp the concept of a advanced detox sunset and amplify it into the night. Restrain exposure to screens, as the harsh artificial light can meddled with melatonin generation. Instep, elect tender, surrounding lighting to form a peaceful environment.

Moon Greetings:
Consolidate an arrangement of yoga postures known as "moon greetings" into your nighttime schedule. These tender and streaming developments can serve as a careful and physical expression of appreciation for the night and its tranquility.

The Effect on Rest Quality:
Grasping nighttime mindfulness not as it were upgrades the quality of the waking minutes but too emphatically impacts rest. By developing a sense of calm and nearness some time recently sleep time, people can encounter moved forward rest onset and a more tranquil night's rest. The move from the quietness of

moonlit mindfulness to the grasp of rest makes an agreeable cadence, supporting in general well-being.

Conclusion:

In a world that frequently appears persistently fast-paced, incorporating moonlit mindfulness offers an asylum of stillness and contemplation. The night, with its firmament ponders and serene climate, gives a canvas for people to develop their association with the display minute and feed their internal selves. By grasping the advantageous relationship between the moon and mindfulness, people can tap into a wellspring of tranquility, advancing mental clarity, passionate adjust, and a significant sense of association to the world around them. Moonlit mindfulness is an welcome to delay, reflect, and appreciate the magnificence of the night "an immortal hone that resounds with the human spirit's require for peace and consideration.

Chapter 7:
Bedtime Sanctuary:
Crafting Your Sleep Oasis

Presentation:

Within the journey for by and large well-being, the significance of quality rest cannot be exaggerated. As the world gets to be progressively fast-paced and interconnected, making a "Sleep time Haven" has developed as a pivotal hone to cultivate tranquil rest and revival. This article investigates the centrality of a rest desert spring, the effect of the rest environment on rest quality, and commonsense steps to plan a sleep time asylum that advances tranquility and unwinding.

Understanding the Significance of Rest:

Quality rest is foundational to physical wellbeing, mental well-being, and cognitive work. Satisfactory and serene rest contributes to the body's repair and recovery, upgrades memory solidification, and underpins passionate strength. In differentiate; destitute rest has been connected to a horde of wellbeing issues, counting expanded push, impaired immune work, and a better chance of incessant conditions.

The Rest Environment's Role:

Making an ideal rest environment could be a key figure in accomplishing helpful rest. The rest environment includes components such as lighting, clamor levels, room temperature, and the generally climate of the room. A well-crafted rest desert spring serves as an asylum that signals to the intellect and body that it's time to loosen up and get ready for a serene night's rest.

Comfortable Bedding:
The establishment of a rest desert garden starts with comfortable bedding. Contribute in high-quality pads, a steady sleeping pad, and delicate, breathable sheets. The material encounter of slipping into a comfortable bed sets the tone for unwinding.

Mindful Lighting:
Light plays a vital part in directing the body's circadian cadence. Dim the lights within the evening to flag to the body that it's time to wind down. Consider utilizing warm-toned, delicate lighting, such as bedside lights or string lights, to form a relieving environment.

Calming Colors:
The color palette of the room can essentially affect the seen climate. Prefer calming and impartial colors, such as delicate blues, quieted greens, or delicate soil tones. These colors contribute to a peaceful environment conducive to unwinding.

Declutter Your Space:
A clutter-free environment advances a sense of calm. Clear superfluous things from surfaces, keep bedside tables clean, and make a sense of arrange within the room. A rearranged space makes a difference calm the intellect and cultivates a quiet environment.

Nature-Inspired Components:
Joining nature-inspired components into the room upgrades the rest desert spring experience. Consider

including pruned plants, characteristic materials, or nature-themed work of art. These components inspire an association to the outside and contribute to a relieving environment.

Fragrance based treatment:
Saddle the control of fragrance based treatment to make a sensory-rich rest environment. Lavender, chamomile, and eucalyptus are known for their calming properties. Utilize fundamental oil diffusers, cloth splashes, or scented candles to implant the room with unwinding scents.

Clamor Lessening:
Minimize troublesome commotions that will meddled with rest. Utilize white clamor machines, earplugs, or noise-canceling gadgets to form a calm environment. On the other hand, consider joining calming sounds, such as delicate precipitation or sea waves, to advance unwinding.

Temperature Control:
Keeping up a comfortable room temperature is fundamental for quality rest. Alter the indoor regulator to a cool, comfortable level, and contribute in breathable bedding materials. Finding the ideal temperature for your rest inclinations contributes to a more relaxing night.

Personalized Decor:
Imbue the rest desert spring with individual touches that bring bliss and consolation. Show cherished photos, consolidate significant work of art, or use decorative elements that resound together with your inclinations.

Personalized decor includes a sense of recognition and warmth to the space.

Technology-Free Zone:
Make a technology-free zone inside the sleep desert spring. Expel screens, counting smartphones, tablets, and toss, from the room. The blue light transmitted by screens can disrupt melatonin generation, making it harder to drop snoozing. Instep, prioritize calming exercises such as perusing a book or practicing unwinding strategies some time recently sleep time.

The Customs of Sleep time Haven:

Set up a Wind-Down Schedule:
A steady wind-down schedule signals to the body that it's time to move into rest. Lock in in calming exercises such as perusing, tender extending, or practicing mindfulness contemplation. Setting up a custom makes an unsurprising arrangement that primes the intellect for rest.

Constrain Stimulants some time recently Bed:
Maintain a strategic distance from expending stimulants such as caffeine or nicotine within the hours driving up to sleep time. These substances can meddle with the ability to drop sleeping. Choose decaffeinated teas, warm drain, or home grown mixtures to advance unwinding.

Make a Rest Plan:
Consistency is key to directing the body's internal clock. Set up a customary rest plan by planning to bed and waking up at the same time each day, indeed on ends of the week. This hone makes a difference adjust the

body's circadian beat and advances a more tranquil rest design.

Careful Breathing Works out:
Join careful breathing works out into the sleep time schedule. Profound, moderate breaths flag to the body that it's time to unwind and loosen up. Procedures such as diaphragmatic breathing or dynamic muscle unwinding can be compelling in advancing a sense of calm.

Utilize Unwinding Procedures:
Test with different unwinding procedures to discover what works best for you. Dynamic muscle unwinding, guided symbolism, or delicate yoga extends can be coordinates into the sleep time schedule to discharge pressure and advance unwinding.

Contribute in Rest Extras:
Consider the utilize of rest embellishments to upgrade consolation. Weighted covers, power outage shades, or rest covers can contribute to making a perfect rest environment tailored to person inclinations.

The Effect on Rest Quality:
Planning a sleep time haven isn't fair a tasteful endeavor; it directly influences sleep quality and by and large well-being. The deliberateness creation of a rest desert garden communicates to the intellect that sleep time may be a sacrosanct time for rest and rejuvenation. Quality rest, encouraged by a thoughtfully made rest environment, contributes to move forward temperament, expanded vitality levels, and upgraded cognitive work.

Conclusion:

Within the hustle and haste of everyday life, the room ought to serve as a safe house for rest and rebuilding. Making a sleep time asylum is an speculation in self-care and an acknowledgment of the significance of quality rest in in general well-being. By paying consideration to the tactile components, climate, and individual inclinations that contribute to a relaxing rest environment, people can make a rest desert spring that advances tranquility and unwinding. Within the grasp of a well-crafted sleep time asylum, the travel into the domain of rest gets to be a custom of self-care and a pathway to waking up revived and prepared to confront the day ahead.

Chapter No 8:
Serenity Asana: Yoga's Embrace Before Lights Out

Presentation:

As the requests of advanced life escalating, finding comfort and tranquility some time recently sleep time has gotten to be progressively fundamental for by and large well-being. Within the interest of a tranquil night's rest, people are turning to the old hone of yoga as a door to tranquility. "Tranquility Asana" typifies the thought of joining yoga into the evening schedule, making a careful and calming pre-sleep custom. This article investigates the centrality of yoga in advancing unwinding, the science behind its effect on rest, and commonsense ways to grasp tranquility asana for a more serene move into the night.

The Interaction of Yoga and Unwinding:
Yoga, originating from antiquated India, isn't fair a physical work out but an all-encompassing approach to harmonizing the intellect, body, and soul. Joining yoga into the sleep time schedule can be a capable instrument for advancing unwinding, facilitating pressure, and planning the body and intellect for a night of helpful rest. The hone of "asana" or yoga stances, combined with careful breathing and reflection, makes a peaceful asana arrangement that serves as a bridge to tranquility.

Calming Physical Pressure:
The different yoga postures target particular muscle bunches, discharging collected pressure and stretch

from the day. Tender stretches and postures offer assistance to reduce snugness within the neck, shoulders, and lower back, regions commonly influenced by the inactive nature of cutting edge ways of life.

Calming the Apprehensive Framework:
Careful breathing, a principal viewpoint of yoga, actuates the parasympathetic anxious framework, moreover known as the "rest and process" framework. This actuation checks the impacts of the thoughtful apprehensive framework, capable for the body's push reaction, actuating a state of calm and unwinding.

Upgrading Mind-Body Mindfulness:
The mindful and think nature of yoga energizes people to be display within the minute, cultivating increased mind-body mindfulness. By interfacing with the breath and centering on the sensations of each posture, specialists can develop a sense of mindfulness that expands into the sleep time schedule.

Logical Experiences into Yoga and Rest:
Various consider have investigated the relationship between yoga and rest, highlighting the positive affect of normal hone on rest quality and term. The taking after logical bits of knowledge shed light on how yoga contributes to a tranquil night's rest:

Directing the Circadian Cadence:
The hone of yoga has been connected to the control of the circadian cadence, the bodies inside clock that oversees the sleep-wake cycle. A think about distributed within the Diary of Clinical Brain research found that reliable yoga hone can contribute to a more

synchronized and adjusted circadian cadence, driving to progressed rest designs.

Decreasing A sleeping disorder Side effects:
A sleeping disorder characterized by trouble falling or remaining sleeping, can be lightened through customary yoga hone. An orderly survey distributed within the diary Rest Pharmaceutical Surveys concluded that yoga is effective in lessening sleep deprivation indications, progressing rest effectiveness, and advancing in general rest quality.

Overseeing Push and Uneasiness:
Persistent push and uneasiness are noteworthy supporters to rest unsettling influences. Yoga's accentuation on unwinding methods, such as profound breathing and reflection, has been appeared to diminish levels of push hormones and advance a sense of calm. Investigate within the Diary of Clinical Brain research shows that yoga-based intercessions are useful for overseeing stress-related rest unsettling influences.

Moving forward Rest Engineering:
The physical stances of yoga, combined with breath control, have been related with enhancements in rest architecture "the in general structure and design of rest cycles. A consider within the Universal Diary of Yoga Treatment found that a standard yoga hone can improve the different stages of rest, driving to a more adjusted and remedial rest encounter.

Viable Steps for Grasping Tranquility Asana:

Make a Quiet Space:

Assign a serene and clutter-free range in your domestic for your sleep time yoga hone. Dim the lights, utilize calming colors, and consolidate components like candles or basic oils to enhance the quietness of the space.

Select Delicate Poses:
Pick for tender and therapeutic yoga postures that advance unwinding instead of energetic and energizing groupings. Postures such as Child's Posture, Legs up the Divider, and Leaning back Butterfly are ideal for winding down some time recently rest.

Center on Breath Mindfulness:
Careful breathing could be a foundation of yoga and an effective apparatus for unwinding. Join profound, diaphragmatic breathing into your asana sequence, permitting each breath to be moderate, consider, and associated with the development of your body.

Incorporate Delicate Extending:
Tender extending makes a difference discharge physical pressure collected amid the day. Center on zones inclined to snugness, such as the neck, shoulders, and hips. Stream through postures that energize a continuous discharge of muscle pressure.

Careful Contemplation:
Conclude your quietness asana hone with a brief careful contemplation. This seems include sitting in a comfortable position, centering on your breath, and tenderly diverting your consideration to the display minute in the event that your intellect starts to meander.

Set up a Steady Schedule:
Consistency is key when joining yoga into your bedtime schedule. Point to hone tranquility asana at the same time each night to flag to your body that it's time to wind down and plan for rest.

Test with Yoga Nitra:
Yoga Nitra, too known as yogic rest, could be a guided contemplation that actuates a state of profound unwinding. Consider consolidating a brief Yoga Nitra session into your sleep time schedule to improve the calming impacts of your tranquility asana hone.

Conclusion:

In the interest of a quiet and tranquil night's rest, the integration of yoga into the sleep time schedule stands as an effective and available hone. Quietness asana typifies the substance of yoga as an instrument for unwinding, stretch decrease, and improved mind-body mindfulness. Logical investigate underpins the positive affect of yoga on rest, making it an important expansion to the weapons store of techniques for advancing sound rest propensities.

By making a sleep time haven through tranquility asana, people can make an agreeable move from the requests of the day to the quietness of the night. The deliberateness and careful hone of yoga some time recently lights out offers not as it were physical benefits but to a mental and enthusiastic refuge an opportunity to let go of the day's stressors and grasp the stillness that clears the way for a restoring night's rest. Within the quietude of quietness asana, people can discover a way to not as it were way better rest but too to a more profound association with their internal selves and the serene pith of the show minute.

Chapter 9:
Mindful Slumber: Nourishing the Inner Self

Presentation:

Within the fast-paced present day world, where stretch and diversions proliferate, the journey for serene and restoring rest has ended up more pivotal than ever. The concept of "Careful Sleep" rises above the conventional approach to sleep time, emphasizing the significance of sustaining the inward self some time recently entering the domain of dreams. This article investigates the importance of careful rest hones, the transaction between mindfulness and the quality of sleep, and commonsense techniques to form a sleep time schedule that cultivates genuine inward food.

Understanding Careful Sleep:

Careful sleep goes past the insignificant act of resting; it typifies a holistic approach to sleep time that coordinating mindfulness hones to make a peaceful and feeding environment for the inward self. It includes the deliberateness development of mindfulness, unwinding, and a profound association with one's inward contemplations and feelings some time recently surrendering to rest.

The Transaction between Mindfulness and Rest Quality:

Push Lessening:

Mindfulness, with its center on the present minute, has been demonstrated to decrease push and uneasiness. As stretch could be a common disruptor of rest, consolidating careful hones some time recently sleep time can make a mental and enthusiastic space conducive to unwinding.

Progressed Rest Onset:
The calming impacts of mindfulness can offer assistance people move easily from alertness to rest. By locks in in careful exercises, such as reflection or delicate extending, the intellect starts to loosen up, clearing the way for a more easy passage into sleep.

Improved Rest Quality:
Mindfulness has been connected to advancements in rest quality, counting expanded term of profound rest and decreased occasions of waking amid the night. This recommends that the deliberateness development of mindfulness can emphatically affect the in general rest involvement.

Passionate Direction:
Careful sleep includes recognizing and grasping one's feelings without judgment. By developing enthusiastic mindfulness and direction some time recently sleep time; people can make a steadier passionate establishment for a quiet night's rest.

Viable Methodologies for Careful Sleep:

Pre-Sleep Contemplation:
Lock in in a brief contemplation session some time recently sleep time to calm the intellect and advance unwinding. Center on the breath, permitting considerations to come and go without connection. There are different guided contemplation apps or recordings particularly outlined for rest that can be joined into the schedule.

Body Filter Unwinding:
Hone a body filter unwinding method to discharge pressure and advance a sense of calm. Beginning from the toes and steadily moving up to the head, bring consideration to each portion of the body, deliberately discharging any zones of snugness or inconvenience.

Careful Breathing Works out:
Join careful breathing works out into your sleep time schedule. Methods such as diaphragmatic breathing or the 4-7-8 method can be successful in advancing unwinding and planning the body for rest.

Journaling:
Devote a couple of minutes to journaling some time recently turning in for the night. Reflect on the day, express appreciation, and discharge any waiting contemplations or concerns onto paper. This hone can offer assistance declutters the intellect and make a sense of closure some time recently rest.

Yoga for Sleep time:
Investigate delicate and helpful yoga postures that are particularly planned for sleep time. This may incorporate forward folds, delicate turns, and unwinding extends that offer assistance discharge physical pressure and advance a sense of ease.

Computerized Detox Sunset:
Extend the concept of a advanced detox nightfall into careful sleep. Constrain screen time at slightest an hour some time recently bed, as the blue light radiated by electronic gadgets can interfere with melatonin generation. Instep, want exercises that advance

unwinding, such as perusing a physical book or tuning in to calming music.

Fragrance based treatment:
Saddle the control of fragrances to make a alleviating rest environment. Lavender, chamomile, and ylang-ylang are known for their calming properties. Join basic oils, sachets, or a diffuser to implant the room with these unwinding fragrances.

Create a Sleep Haven:
Change your room into a safe house of tranquility. Select calming colors, contribute in comfortable bedding, and minimize clutter. Making a rest haven upgrades the by and large air and fortifies the thought of bedtime as a sacrosanct and serene time.

Dynamic Muscle Unwinding:
Dynamically tense and after that unwind diverse muscle bunches within the body. Beginning from the toes and moving up to the head, this strategy makes a difference discharge physical pressure, advancing a sense of unwinding and planning the body for rest.

Appreciation Hone:
Develop a sense of appreciation some time recently sleep time by reflecting on positive perspectives of the day. This hone shifts center from potential stressors to positive encounters, cultivating a more positive and serene attitude conducive to rest.

Benefits of Careful Sleep:
Upgraded Well-being:
Careful sleep contributes to in general well-being by advancing unwinding, diminishing push, and cultivating

a positive mentality. Quality rest is naturally connected to physical and mental wellbeing, making careful sleep a basic component of a sound way of life.

Moved forward Cognitive Work:
Satisfactory and serene rest is significant for cognitive work. Careful sleep bolsters cognitive forms, counting memory combination, problem-solving, and decision-making, driving to make strides mental clarity and center amid waking hours.

Enthusiastic Strength:
Mindfulness hones some time recently sleep time develops passionate strength by advancing mindfulness and acknowledgment of feelings. This strength can contribute to a more adjusted and steady enthusiastic state, lessening the probability of passionate unsettling influences amid rest.

Fortified Mind-Body Association:
Locks in in careful sleep strengthens the mind-body association. By deliberately going to to the body and intellect some time recently rest, people can extend their understanding of the interconnecting between physical sensations, thoughts, and emotions.

Conclusion:
In a world that frequently commends busyness and efficiency, the esteem of careful sleep could be a tender update of the significance of self-care and inward food. Past the mechanical act of rest, careful sleep welcomes people to approach sleep time as a sacrosanct and deliberateness practice a time to discharge the day's burdens, grasp internal stillness, and cultivate a significant association with oneself. By joining

mindfulness into the sleep time schedule, people can tap into the transformative control of sleep, opening not as it were physical rebuilding but moreover passionate and otherworldly recharging. Careful sleep is a welcome to set out on a daily travel of self-discovery, flexibility, and the calm grasp of internal peace.

Chapter 10:
Workday Release: Yoga for Stress Resilience
Presentation:

Within the hustle and flurry of the modern work environment, where requests are tall and the weight to perform is consistent, stretch has gotten to be an unwelcome companion for numerous experts. The journey for successful methodologies to oversee and ease stretch has driven to a worldview move, with "Workday Discharge: Yoga for Stretch Strength" developing as a transformative approach. This article investigates the significant effect of yoga on push flexibility, digs into the science behind the mind-body association, and gives down to earth experiences on consistently consolidating yoga into the workday for improved well-being and efficiency.

Understanding the Inescapable Nature of Working environment Stretch:

Workplace stretch may be an omnipresent marvel in today's fast-paced proficient world. The tireless requests of due dates, obligations, and the inescapable impact of innovation have made an environment where push can raise quickly. The results of unmanaged push expand past the mental domain, showing physically and influencing in general well-being. Recognizing the require for proactive stretch administration is foremost to cultivating a more advantageous work-life adjust.

The Science of Yoga and Push Versatility:
Mind-Body Association:

Yoga, established in old hones, flourishes on the rule of cultivating an agreeable mind-body association.

Through the combination of breath work, reflection, and physical stances, yoga develops increased mindfulness of the show minute. This complicated association gets to be a capable instrument in overseeing stretch, empowering people to watch stressors with more noteworthy strength and react more successfully.

Push Diminishment Hormones:
Locks in in yoga triggers the discharge of stress-reducing hormones, such as cortisol. The energetic combination of controlled breathing and purposefulness development makes a difference direct cortisol levels, introducing in a sense of calm and unwinding. By consistently joining yoga into the workday, people can proactively oversee their push reactions.

Advancing the Unwinding Reaction:
The hone of yoga enacts the parasympathetic anxious framework, frequently alluded to as the "rest and process" framework. This enactment counterbalances the physiological impacts of the "battle or flight" reaction initiated by stretch. As a result, heart rate brings down, blood pressure reduces, and a unavoidable sense of calmness follows, cultivating flexibility within the confront of stressors.

Progressed Passionate Direction:
Mindfulness, a center component of yoga, upgrades passionate control. By developing mindfulness of contemplations and sentiments without judgment, people create the devices to explore stressors more viably. Emotional resilience, supported through yoga,

deciphers into a more adjusted and composed reaction to challenges within the working environment.

Upgraded Cognitive Work:
Yoga has been logically connected to moved forward cognitive work. The hone, which envelops contemplation and mindfulness, upgrades consideration, concentration, and memory. Given that stretch can disable cognitive execution, joining yoga into the workday underpins mental sharpness and efficiency.

Commonsense Integration of Yoga into the Workday:
Work area Yoga:
Begin with work area yoga, consolidating brief arrangements that discharge pressure and advance adaptability. Straightforward extends, neck and bear rolls, and situated turns can be cautiously performed at the work area, offering instant alleviation amid the workday.

Breath work Breaks:
Plan brief breaks all through the day for deliberateness breath work. Profound, diaphragmatic breathing or "pranayama" can be practiced in a calm corner or indeed at the work area. Coordinating consideration to the breath encourages a centering impact, lightening stretch.

Careful Minutes:
Coordinated brief minutes of mindfulness into the workday. Whether it's a five-minute guided reflection amid a break or a careful walk around the office, these

minutes divert consideration to the show and contribute to stretch flexibility.

Lunchtime Yoga Sessions:
Companies are progressively recognizing the benefits of on-site yoga classes or dedicating a space for representatives to hone amid lunch breaks. This offers a restoring break from work-related stressors and cultivates a more positive work environment culture.

Chair Yoga:
Chair yoga is an available and helpful way to coordinated yoga into the workday. Situated extends, turns, and tender developments can be done cautiously at the work area, catering to people with restricted versatility or a desk-bound schedule.

Virtual Yoga Classes:
Use innovation to get to virtual yoga classes or apps advertising guided sessions. This adaptability permits workers to lock in in yoga from the consolation of their workspace or amid assigned breaks, making the hone more available.

Assembly Mindfulness:
Start or conclude gatherings with a brief mindfulness work out. This may well be a brief contemplation, a careful breathing work out, or a collective extend to neutralize the impacts of drawn out sitting and implant a sense of calm into the work environment.

Assigned Unwinding Spaces:
Make devoted spaces inside the working environment where representatives can withdraw for minutes of unwinding and yoga hone. Prepared with yoga mats and

calming stylistic layout, these spaces serve as havens for restoration in the midst of the requests of the work environment.

Stress-Relieving Postures:
Join stress-relieving yoga postures into the workday schedule. Postures such as Child's Posture, Forward Overlap, and Legs Up the Divider can be done independently or as portion of a brief yoga sequence to lighten pressure and advance unwinding.

Instructive Workshops:
Have workshops on push versatility and the benefits of yoga for representatives. Bringing in yoga teaches or wellness specialists to lead sessions cannot as it were teach workers but moreover cultivate a culture of well-being inside the work environment.

Benefits of Yoga for Stretch Strength:
Expanded Strength:
A normal yoga hone enhances resilience by giving people with compelling apparatuses to manage with stressors. The mindfulness developed in yoga engages people to explore challenges with a adjusted and composed mentality.

Made strides Physical Well-being:
Yoga contributes to physical well-being by lightening solid pressure, improving adaptability, and advancing superior pose. Tending to the physical toll of push on the body comes about in diminished side effects such as back torment and migraines.

Upgraded Center and Efficiency:

The made strides cognitive work coming about from yoga interprets into heightened center and efficiency. Representatives who lock in in yoga are superior prepared to preserve concentration and perform successfully in requesting work circumstances.

Positive Working environment Culture:
Consolidating yoga into the workday cultivates a positive working environment culture that values representative well-being. This may lead to expanded work fulfillment, moved forward worker maintenance, and the foundation of a more concordant work environment.

Passionate Well-being:
Yoga promotes passionate well-being by giving a space for people to associate with and direct their feelings. The mindfulness hones inserted in yoga contribute

Chapter 11:
Presentation:

Rest may be an essential perspective of human well-being, playing a significant part in physical wellbeing, mental flexibility, and by and large efficiency. In a world characterized by consistent network and boisterous plans, building up a serene schedule has ended up more challenging however more basic than ever. This article investigates the significance of rest, the science behind it, and viable procedures for building a strong establishment for tranquil evenings.

I. Understanding the Significance of Sleep:
Organic Noteworthiness:

Rest may be a complex organic handle that includes different stages, each serving a special reason. It is during sleep that the body experiences pivotal repairs, and the brain solidifies recollections. Disappointment to urge satisfactory rest can disable cognitive work, debilitate the safe framework, and contribute to different wellbeing issues.

Effect on Mental Wellbeing:

The relationship between rest and mental wellbeing is significant. Need of rest has been connected to expanded stretch, uneasiness, and discouragement. Alternately, prioritizing quality sleep can improve enthusiastic versatility, temperament solidness, and in general mental well-being.

Physical Rebuilding:

Rest could be a time for the body to mend and reestablish itself. Cellular repair, muscle development, and the discharge of development hormones transcendently happen amid the more profound stages of rest. A steady need of rest can compromise physical wellbeing and ruin the body's capacity to recoup from day by day stressors.

II. The Science of Rest:
Circadian Rhythms:

Our bodies work on a circadian cadence, a normal inside clock that controls the sleep-wake cycle. Understanding and adjusting with this beat is significant for optimizing the quality of rest. Introduction to common light amid the day and making a dim, calm environment at night offer assistance control these rhythms.

Rest Engineering:

Rest is partitioned into a few cycles, counting REM (Fast Eye Development) and non-REM stages. Each organize serves particular capacities, contributing to by and large rest quality. Building up a schedule that permits for adequate time in each arrange is basic for a tranquil night's rest.

Rest Cleanliness:

Rest cleanliness envelops hones and propensities that advance sound rest. This incorporates keeping up a steady rest plan, making a comfortable rest environment, and dodging stimulants like caffeine near to sleep time. These hones contribute to the in general quality of rest.

III. Building a Tranquil Rest Schedule:
Building up Steady Rest Designs:

Making a normal rest plan makes a difference direct the body's inner clock. Planning to bed and waking up at the same time each day, indeed on ends of the week, strengthens the circadian beat, making it simpler to drop sleeping and wake up normally.

Making a Unwinding Sleep time Schedule:
Locks in in calming exercises some time recently sleep time signals to the body that it's time to wind down. This may incorporate exercises such as perusing a book, taking a warm shower, or practicing unwinding strategies like profound breathing or contemplation.

Optimizing the Rest Environment:
The room environment plays a significant role in rest quality. Keeping the room cool, dull, and calm makes an ideal setting for rest. Contributing in a comfortable sleeping pad and pads that bolster legitimate spinal arrangement is additionally pivotal.

Restricting Screen Time:
Introduction to the blue light transmitted by screens can meddle with the body's generation of melatonin, a hormone that controls rest. Setting up a computerized check in time and maintaining a strategic distance from screens at slightest an hour some time recently sleep time can contribute to a more tranquil rest.

Directing Nourishment and Drink Admissions:
Expending overwhelming suppers, caffeine, and liquor near to sleep time can disturb rest. Selecting for a light nibble on the off chance that hungry and remaining hydrated with water are ideal evening choices to bolster relaxing rest.

Standard Physical Action:
Customary work out has been appeared to progress rest quality. Locks in in physical movement prior within the day can offer assistance direct rest designs and advance a more profound, more remedial rest.

Stretch Administration:
Tall push levels can meddle with the capacity to relax and drop sleeping. Consolidating stress-reducing hones such as mindfulness, yoga, or journaling into the evening schedule can be advantageous for advancing a calm state of intellect some time recently sleep time.

Conclusion:
Building a relaxing rest schedule may be a multifaceted handle that includes understanding the science of rest, prioritizing its importance, and receiving down to earth methodologies to bolster solid rest propensities. By joining these components into existence, people can lay the establishment for tranquil evenings, eventually contributing to made strides physical and mental well-being. In a world that frequently commends busyness, contributing within the time and exertion to sustain a sound rest schedule could be a capable act of self-care with far-reaching benefits .Sleep Foundations: Building a Restful Routine

Chapter 12:
Desk to Dreamland: Seamless Evening Transitions
Presentation:

As the day winds down, the move from work to rest gets to be a significant period for setting the arrange for a tranquil night's rest. The cutting edge way of life, regularly characterized by requesting work plans and consistent network, can make this move challenging. Be that as it may, actualizing a consistent evening schedule can bridge the hole between a boisterous day at the work area and a relaxing night in fairyland. This article dives into the significance of evening moves, the science behind winding down, and commonsense methodologies to form a concordant bridge between the workdays and sleep time.

I. Recognizing the Significance of Evening Moves:
Circadian Rhythms and Move Signals:

The human body works on a characteristic circadian beat, a 24-hour inner clock that controls the sleep-wake cycle. Making unmistakable signals for the body to recognize the move from work to unwinding makes a difference synchronize with these rhythms. Building up steady evening moves upgrades the body's capacity to wind down and plan for a relaxing night.

Effect on Rest Quality:

The quality of evening moves straightforwardly impacts the consequent rest quality. Locks in in calming exercises and making a conducive environment amid the move period signals to the body that it's time to unwind. This, in turn, advances the discharge of sleep-inducing hormones and cultivates a more profound, more remedial rest.

II. The Science of Winding Down:
Melatonin and Rest Hormones:

Melatonin, regularly alluded to as the "rest hormone," plays a significant part in controlling the sleep-wake cycle. Introduction to common light during the day and haziness within the evening fortifies melatonin generation. By understanding and leveraging this hormone, people can optimize their evening moves for superior rest.

Blue Light and Rest Disturbance:

Electronic gadgets emanate blue light, which can meddled with melatonin generation and disrupt the sleep-wake cycle. Minimizing screen time, particularly within the hour driving up to sleep time, makes a difference moderate these impacts and bolsters a smoother move to rest.

III. Down to earth Procedures for Consistent Evening Moves:
Characterize a Clear Conclusion to the Workday:

Physically and rationally stamping the conclusion of the workday is fundamental for making a boundary between proficient and individual life. This might include closing down the computer, turning off work-related notices, and making a typical end-of-day schedule to flag the move.

Lock in in Unwinding Exercises:

Transitioning from work to rest can be encouraged by locks in in calming exercises. Perusing a book, practicing delicate extending or yoga, or tuning in to relieving music are viable ways to flag to the body that it's time to loosen up.

Make a Comfortable Environment:
The room environment altogether impacts rest quality. Making the bed, diminishing lights, and altering the room temperature contribute to a cozy and welcoming climate, advancing unwinding and signaling the move to rest.

Computerized Detox:
Constraining presentation to screens, particularly those emanating blue light is vital for a consistent evening move. Setting up a computerized detox schedule within the hour some time recently sleep time permits the intellect to separate from the requests of the day and bolsters the body's normal wind-down prepare.

Mindfulness and Unwinding Procedures:
Consolidating mindfulness hones, such as profound breathing works out or reflection, into the evening schedule can be instrumental in calming the intellect. These strategies advance unwinding, diminish push, and encourage a smoother move into a tranquil state.

Progressive Decompression:
Instep of unexpectedly finishing work-related assignments, slowly winding down can make the move more consistent. Prioritize assignments, total a to-do list, and rationally plan for the following day. This makes a difference make a sense of closure and minimizes waiting work-related contemplations.

Hydrate Mindfully:

Whereas remaining hydrated are basic, expending huge amounts of liquids right some time recently sleep time can disturb rest due to visit trips to the washroom. Hydrating mindfully, by decreasing off liquid admissions an hour some time recently rest, guarantees ideal hydration without compromising rest.

Conclusion:

A consistent move from the work area to never land is a speculation in in general well-being. Recognizing the significance of evening moves, understanding the science behind winding down, and executing viable procedures can change the way people approach sleep time. By prioritizing this move, people can develop a serene environment that not as it were progresses rest quality but too contributes to improved efficiency and mental well-being amid waking hours. From characterizing clear boundaries at the conclusion of the workday to locks in in unwinding exercises, each step plays a crucial role in making a agreeable bridge between the requests of the day and the tranquility of the night.

Chapter 13:
Nitra Nurturing: Deep Yogic Sleep Exploration
First of all,

Yoga, an age-old discipline dedicated to the quest of comprehensive well-being, has a transforming effect on sleep in addition to physical postures and breath control. Often called "yogic sleep" or "psychic sleep," yoga nitro is a profound practice that uses awareness, relaxation, and meditation techniques to help people enter a deep, conscious sleep. This article explores the foundational ideas and advantages of Yoga Nitra, as well as the history, scientific basis, and doable implementation strategies for this restorative practice in everyday life.

I. An Overview of Yoga Nitra:
Origin and Roots:

The Tantras, in particular, are the source of yoga Nida's ancient yogic traditions. Although the word "Nitra" means sleep, the practice extends beyond simple slumber. It entails a condition of conscious relaxation in which the body is at rest and the mind is awake. Midway through the 20th century, Swami Stay Ananda Sarasvati—a pivotal person in the practice of Yoga Nitra—introduced it as a methodical approach.

The Basics of Yoga Nidra:

Essentially, Yoga Nidra is a guided meditation that progresses a person through many levels of relaxation until they reach a profound state of calm. Yoga Nidra promotes a level of alertness and elevated consciousness as the body undergoes profound relaxation, in contrast to conventional sleep, where the mind may drift into dreams.

II. **Yoga Nitra's Science Basis:**
Brain Wave States:

Practicing yoga nitro causes a transition in brain waves from the beta state of waking to the alpha stage of relaxation and, finally, the theta state of profound sleep. This shift eases tension, encourages rest, and makes it easier for the conscious and subconscious minds to communicate.

Parasympathetic Dominance:

Often known as the "rest and digest" system, the technique stimulates the parasympathetic nervous system. This approach encourages rest, decreases heart rate, and strengthens the body's capacity for renewal and repair.

Cortisol Regulation and Stress Reduction:

Yoga Nidra has been associated with lower cortisol levels, which are a measure of stress. By reducing stress, the practice enhances general well-being, improves mental health, and improves the quality of sleep.

III. **Yoga Nitra's Advantages**
Improved Sleep Quality:

Yoga Nidra is a potent method for enhancing the quality of sleep because it induces deep relaxation that develops a profound sensation of peace. Yoga Nidra is a useful technique for people who have trouble sleeping or are restless at night.

Stress Reduction and Anxiety Management:

Yoga Nidra is a powerful practice for reducing stress and managing tension and anxiety. Frequent practice develops inner tranquility, which acts as a defense against the stresses of everyday life.

Enhanced Cognitive performance:
During Yoga Nidra, conscious awareness is maintained, which improves cognitive performance. The exercise helps with decision-making, problem-solving, and general mental sharpness by promoting attention and clarity.

Mind-Body Connection:
Yoga Nidra helps to establish a strong mental-physical bond. During the practice, people develop a heightened awareness of physical sensations by focusing on different regions of their bodies, which fosters a sense of unity and well-being.

Resilience and Emotional Healing:
Yoga Nidra offers a space for emotional processing and healing. People can increase their emotional resilience and adopt a more balanced approach to situations by admitting and letting go of pent-up feelings.

IV. Applying Yoga Nidra to Everyday Situations: Developing a Consistent Practice:
To really benefit from Yoga Nidra, like with any transformative practice, consistency is essential. Establishing a habit and developing a stronger bond with the practice can be facilitated by setting aside specific time each day, whether it be in the morning or right before bed.

Establishing a Sacred environment:

Making an environment that is calm and cozy for the practice improves it all around. A comfortable blanket, soft couches, and dim lighting all help create a calm atmosphere that is ideal for unwinding.

Making Use of Guided Recordings:
Guided recordings of Yoga Nidra are quite helpful for those who are new to it. It is possible for people of all skill levels to receive guided sessions conducted by seasoned practitioners using a variety of media, including as applications, websites, and audio recordings.
Prior to every Yoga Nidra session, establishing a clear goal, or sankalpa, amplifies the practice's transformational potential. Whether the goal is to solve a particular issue, foster self-love, or develop gratitude, a well-defined intention directs the subconscious mind in the direction of good development.

Combining with Asana and Pranayama:
The overall advantages of Yoga Nidra are increased when it is incorporated into a more comprehensive yoga practice that incorporates physical postures (asana) and breath control (pranayama). Together, they provide a comprehensive strategy for well-being that takes into account mental, spiritual, and bodily aspects.

In summary:
A profound doorway to deeper rest and regeneration is yoga nitro. This ancient practice provides a haven for people who want to develop a calm mind, a rested body, and a fed spirit in a fast-paced world full of stressors and unending expectations. People can begin a transforming journey toward holistic well-being and the nurturing embrace of yogic sleep by learning about the

history, science, and advantages of Yoga Nidra and consciously and consistently incorporating it into their daily lives.

Chapter 14:
Sleep Science Unveiled: Understanding Your Rest

Sleep is a complicated physiological and psychological process that has long captivated scientists and academics despite being thought of as a straightforward, passive activity. The study of sleep science is a fast developing discipline that aims to understand the complexities of this essential component of human existence. Through investigating the processes, phases, and outcomes of sleep, researchers are illuminating the ways in which sleep affects our mental, emotional, and physical health.

Every stage of the sleep cycle has a distinct function and is arranged in a symphony by the brain. The two primary stages of sleep, known as REM (rapid eye movement) and non-REM, occur at intervals of approximately 90 to 120 minutes. Physical restoration and deeper relaxation are the hallmarks of non-REM sleep, which is divided into three phases. While sleep is progressively deeper throughout Stages 2 and 3, which support muscle growth, repair, and general physical recovery, Stage 1 signifies the change from waking to sleep.

Restoration of cognition is linked to the REM period, which is also known for vivid dreams. In this phase, memories are solidified, emotions are dealt with, and critical cognitive processes are carried out. For the body's general health and functionality, the complex tango between the REM and non-REM phases is essential.

For the body and mind to operate properly, there must be a balance between the non-REM and REM phases.

Understanding the importance of the body's internal clock, the circadian rhythm, is essential to comprehending sleep. The sleep-wake cycle is influenced by this natural biological cycle, which also controls hormone production, attentiveness, and other vital body processes. The significance of keeping a regular sleep schedule in sync with one's circadian cycle is underscored by the fact that disturbances to this rhythm, including shift work or irregular sleep patterns, can result in sleep disorders and contribute to a host of health problems.

Sleep quality is a crucial component of sleep science, yet it is sometimes overlooked in favor of quantity. Establishing a conducive sleeping environment and implementing good sleep hygiene are necessary for obtaining restorative sleep. The temperature of the room, light exposure, and using electronics right before bed can all have a big impact on how well you sleep. People who prioritize the quality of their sleep over its quantity can benefit from deeper levels of both physical and mental renewal.

Furthermore, studies in the field of sleep science have shed light on the far-reaching consequences of insufficient sleep on general health. Long-term sleep deprivation is linked to a higher risk of diabetes, obesity, and reduced cognitive performance and cardiovascular disease. Insufficient sleep can affect the body's capacity to fight off infections and illnesses because the immune system depends on it as well for healthy functioning. A healthy lifestyle necessitates getting enough sleep, which is made even more important when one considers the wider health ramifications.

Research on sleep has been transformed by technological developments, which have given scholars the means to investigate its secrets with never-before-seen depth. An invaluable diagnostic tool for sleep disorders and patterns is polysomnography, which tracks muscle activity, eye movements, and brain waves as a patient sleeps. Autography is a non-invasive technique for tracking sleep-wake cycles that includes wearing a gadget that tracks movement.
These technological advancements have improved not just our comprehension of sleep but also allowed for more precise diagnosis and focused treatment of sleep problems.

Effects on the body, sleep science explore the complex relationships that exist between sleep and mental and emotional health. For memory consolidation, emotional control, and cognitive performance, adequate sleep is essential. Research has demonstrated that sleep deprivation is linked to anxiety, mental disorders, and a reduced capacity to handle stress. Furthermore, sleep is essential for improving learning and problem-solving skills, which makes it a foundational element of both professional and academic success.

Summary, the field of sleep science has advanced and shed light on one of the most essential human experiences: sleep. The discipline continues to offer important insights into the significance of comprehending and prioritizing sleep, from the regulation of the sleep cycle to the significant ramifications of insufficient rest on physical and mental health. Growing awareness of the wide-ranging effects of sleep deprivation has made society realize how important it is to develop healthy sleep habits and treat sleep disorders. Ultimately, having a thorough understanding of sleep science enables people to make decisions that will ultimately lead to a happier, healthier life.

Chapter 15:
Dream Cuisine: Nighttime Foods for Better Sleep

In our fast-paced world, where stretch and steady movement frequently overwhelm our everyday lives, the journey for superior rest has ended up a need for numerous. Whereas different variables contribute to a great night's rest, counting a conducive rest environment and steady rest schedules, the part of sustenance in advancing solid rest designs is picking up expanding consideration. Enter the domain of "Dream Cooking," a concept that investigates the effect of nighttime nourishments on the quality of our rest.

Understanding the association between slim down and rest requires a closer see at the complicated interaction between certain supplements and the body's sleep-regulating components. Various consider have highlighted the impact of particular nourishments on the generation of sleep-inducing hormones and neurotransmitters. Consolidating the correct nourishments into your evening schedule can contribute to a more tranquil and restoring rest involvement.

One of the key players in advancing superior rest is tryptophan, an amino corrosive that serves as a antecedent to serotonin and melatonin, both vital hormones for controlling rest. Turkey, known for its tall tryptophan substance, has earned its notoriety as a classic Thanksgiving liberality, regularly taken after by a post-feast rest. Be that as it may, tryptophan isn't elite to turkey; other sources incorporate chicken, nuts, seeds, and dairy items.

In expansion to tryptophan, magnesium is another basic supplement connected to made strides rest quality. Magnesium plays a part in directing neurotransmitters that initiate rest and advance muscle unwinding. Nourishments wealthy in magnesium, such as verdant green vegetables, nuts, seeds, and entirety grains, can be advantageous increments to an evening supper or nibble.

The sleep-promoting impacts of certain nourishments expand past their wholesome substance to their capacity to control blood sugar levels. Nourishments with a moo glycemic file discharge glucose slowly, anticipating the fast spikes and crashes that can disturb rest. Entire grains, vegetables, and vegetables are fabulous choices for keeping up steady blood sugar levels all through the night.

Herbs and flavors have moreover been recognized for their potential to improve rest. Chamomile tea, for occurrence, contains cancer prevention agents and compounds that will have a gentle narcotic impact, advancing unwinding. Joining herbs like lavender and valerian into your evening schedule, either through mixtures or as seasonings in your suppers, can contribute to a calming environment conducive to rest. The concept of Dream Food expands past person supplements to the broader thought of making adjusted and feeding dinners that back generally well-being. Maintaining a strategic distance from overwhelming, wealthy, and zesty nourishments near to sleep time is prudent, as these can lead to acid reflux and inconvenience, possibly disturbing rest. Picking for lighter, nutrient-dense alternatives can give the vital food without overpowering the stomach related framework.

Timing plays a significant part in maximizing the benefits of Dream Food. Devouring a well-balanced evening supper around 2-3 hours some time recently sleep time permits for legitimate assimilation and minimizes the chance of distress. Late-night snacking, particularly on sugary or caffeinated nourishments, ought to be drawn nearer with caution, as these can meddled with the body's normal circadian beat and disturb the move into relaxing rest.

Whereas the center is regularly on supper, it's fundamental not to miss the potential effect of sleep time snacks on rest quality. A little, adjusted nibble containing a combination of protein and complex carbohydrates can offer assistance stabilize blood sugar levels and give a delicate discharge of tryptophan all through the night. Greek yogurt with a sprinkle of nuts, a banana with almond butter, or a whole-grain saltine with cheese are all illustrations of bedtime-friendly snacks.

The importance of hydration in advancing superior rest ought to not be belittled. Home grown teas, such as chamomile or valerian, not as it were contribute to the Dream Food concept but moreover offer a relieving and hydrating elective to caffeinated refreshments. Remaining enough hydrated underpins generally wellbeing and can avoid inconvenience amid the night.

In conclusion, Dream Food offers an all-encompassing approach to progressing rest quality through careful nourishment choices and eating propensities. By understanding the effect of particular supplements on sleep-regulating instruments, people can tailor their evening suppers to back tranquil and restoring rest. Joining an assortment of nourishments wealthy in tryptophan, magnesium, and other sleep-promoting compounds, whereas being careful of supper timing and maintaining a strategic distance from troublesome late-night snacks, can contribute to a more quiet night's rest. Grasping the standards of Dream Food not as it were upgrades rest but moreover cultivates a more profound association between sustenance and by and large well-being, clearing the way for a more adjusted and satisfying way of life.

Chapter 16:

Morning Vitality: Yoga Energizers for a Strong Start

Presentation

The way you begin your morning sets the tone for the rest of the day. Consolidating yoga into your morning schedule can be a capable way to stir your body and intellect, advancing essentialness and a positive attitude. In this investigation of morning imperativeness, we dive into the world of yoga energizers that can assist you kick start your day with quality, adaptability, and a sense of inward adjust.

Sun Welcome (Surya Namesake)

One of the foremost well-known and comprehensive yoga arrangements for morning essentialness is the Sun Welcome. Comprising of an arrangement of 12 postures performed in a streaming arrangement, Sun Greetings lock in different muscle bunches and advance adaptability. The dreary nature of the arrangement moreover serves as a moving reflection, making a difference to calm the intellect whereas strengthening the body.

Start by standing at the front of your tangle, breathe in, and raise your arms overhead. Breathe out as you overlay forward, putting your hands on the tangle. Breathe in, lift your chest, and see forward. As you breathe out, step or bounce back into a board position, bringing down into a chattering. Breathe in into an upward-facing dog, breathe out into a downward-facing puppy, and after that step or hop back to the front of the tangle to rehash the arrangement. Point for 5 to 10 rounds, syncing your breath with the developments.

Energizing Breath (Pranayama)

Breath is the substance of life, and saddling its control through pranayama can essentially affect your morning essentialness. Procedures like Kapalbhati (skull-shining breath) and Bhastrika (howls breathe) invigorate the respiratory framework, increment oxygen admissions, and stir the body's vitality.

To hone Kapalbhati, sit comfortably with a straight spine. Breathe in profoundly; at that point mightily breathe out through your nose by contracting your stomach muscles. Permit the inward breathe to happen inactively, centering on the fast and cadenced exhalations. Begin with 1-2 minutes and steadily increment the length as your hone creates.

Cat-Cow Extend (Marjaryasana-Bitilasana)

This delicate, streaming development warms up the spine and locks in the center muscles. Start on your hands and knees, along with your wrists straightforwardly beneath your shoulders and your knees beneath your hips. Breathe in, curve your back, and lift your head and tailbone toward the ceiling (Dairy animals Pose). Exhale, circular your spine, and tuck your chin to your chest (Cat Posture). Stream between these two poses for many minutes, synchronizing your breath with each development.

The Cat-Cow extend not as it were advances adaptability within the spine but too makes a difference discharge pressure and stretch, taking off you feeling more energized and centered.

Warrior Postures (Virabhadrasana I and II)

Channel the quality of a warrior with Virabhadrasana I (Warrior Posture I) and Virabhadrasana II (Warrior

Posture II). These postures construct quality within the legs, open the chest, and make strides center and adjust. To hone Warrior I, begin in a standing position, step one foot back, and turn it at a 45-degree point. Twist the front knee over the lower leg, coming to your arms overhead. Keep your back leg straight and solid, establishing through the external edge of the foot. For Warrior II, amplify your arms parallel to the floor, with the front knee still bowed. Look over the front hand and lock in your center. Hold each posture for 30 seconds to a miniature, breathing profoundly and feeling the control and vitality transmit through your body.

Bending Postures (Aroha Matsyendrasana)
Twisting poses offer assistance fortifies assimilation, detoxify the organs, and discharge pressure within the spine. Ardha Matsyendrasana, or Half Ruler of the Fishes Posture, could be a situated turn that energizes the spine and stimulates the stomach related organs. Sit on the floor along with your legs amplified. Twist your right knee and place your foot on the exterior of your cleared out thigh. Breathe in, stretch your spine, and turn to the correct, bringing your cleared out elbow exterior your right knee. Hold the posture for 30 seconds to a diminutive, breathing profoundly and steadily deepening the twist.
Rehash on the other side, permitting the tender turning movement to stir your body and intellect, clearing out you feeling revived and revitalized.

Conclusion

Joining these yoga energizers into your morning schedule can change the way you begin your day. Whether you have got a devoted hour or fair some minutes, these hones offer an all-encompassing approach to morning essentialness, combining physical development, breath work, and mindfulness. By making yoga a reliable portion of your morning schedule, you not as it were improve your physical well-being but moreover develop a positive and centered attitude that can emphatically affect all viewpoints of your day. So, roll out your tangle, take a profound breath, and grasp the control of morning essentialness through yoga.